Japanese Diet:
Easiest Way To Lose 15 Pounds In Two Weeks

Table of content

Introduction

You catch sight of yourself in the mirror as you walk by, and you can't help but sigh. You want to lose weight, you've tried to lose weight, but it seems the more you try, the harder it is to actually lose.

You are tired of being unhappy. You are tired of not liking how you look, you are tired of the way you feel, and you just want it all to go away. But, you don't think you could be happy going vegan, or low carb, or no carb, or even paleo. You like to eat what you like to eat, and those all sound so hard and expensive.

You need a diet that is going to give you the results you are looking for, but isn't going to weigh you down with countless rules and regulations while you get there. You need a diet that is going to give you results, and give them to you quickly.

You need something that works.

Thankfully, you have come to the right place. In this book, you are going to find everything you need to know about the Japanese diet – a diet that is as old as time, and one that works.

Now, the Japanese diet isn't going to be Asian food. Don't think that when you are on this diet you're going to eat a lot of what the Asians do. No, the Japanese diet is so named because of the simplicity of the diet – which is how the Japanese live their lives.

It is highly effective, restricting the calories you put into your body while helping you burn through the extra. You will lose the weight quickly, and you will be able to keep it off. With this diet, you're going to get everything you need to succeed, and this book is going to help you, every step of the way.

Let me show you the secret to this ancient practice, and help you lose weight, feel great, and get to where you want to be – before summer even arrives.

This book is your weight loss hero, and it's going to give you the keys you need to lose weight and keep it off for good. You have finally found the answer to what you have been looking for.

And it's never looked better.

Chapter 1 – So You Want To Lose Weight?

You know you've tried everything, and at this point, you would give anything just to be able to lose some weight. You have been to the gym, you've tried to diets, and you have wanted this more than anything, but it's simply not been happening.

What is the secret to weight loss? How are you going to actually lose the weight when there are so many different (and opposite) diets on the market, telling you to do completely opposite things to make it happen?

Trust me, I understand your situation, because I have been there. But I have also found the secret to losing weight, and I am going to share that with you. With the Japanese diet, you're going to find the weight loss you have been looking for, and fast.

Using the simply method of calories in versus calories out, this diet doesn't get caught up in all the nutritional nonsense. It eliminates salt, alcohol, sugars, and others that are known to hold weight loss back, but it allows you to eat most of the foods you love.

Leaning heavily on rice, this diet tends to cut out as many calories as possible, maximizing your weight loss. With this in mind, you must realize that fast diets do slow your metabolism, and if they are abused, they can potentially do long term damage.

Listen to your body and never starve yourself, and if you have any other medical condition, consult your doctor before you go on the Japanese diet. This diet is going to give you regular meal times, but the meals are small and you won't be snacking in between.

Pay attention to how you feel, and don't be afraid to break the diet if you feel that your blood sugar has dropped further than it should.

Restrict yourself to using this diet only once every six months, and eat as you normally do the rest of the time. Do this, and you're going to see the results you wish to see, and be able to fit into the size clothing you want to fit into. This diet truly is going to give you everything you want, and then some.

So get ready to change your life for the better, and dive into a new world of weight loss that gives you the results you have been looking for. Summer is on the way, and you know what you want to be wearing.

Good luck.

Chapter 2 – Simple Exercises To Boost Your Metabolism

Any weight loss regimen should be accompanied by some form of exercise. Sure, it is possible to lose weight through your diet alone, but when you do that, you risk ruining your metabolism, and ruining any future chance of losing weight the healthy way.

When you lose weight, you should always work in some form of exercise, which is why I have included this simply section here. You don't have to spend hours a day breaking your back at the gym – just a few minutes of your time per day, and you'll find yourself on the right track to a happy and healthy life.

Throughout the next two weeks, make an effort 5 days a week to get your heart rate up for 20 minutes per day. You can do this all at once, or you can break it down into 2, 10 minute sessions.

Take a day off every now and then, but never more than 1 day in a row.

Yoga.

Yoga is a great way to melt off the pounds while getting fit. With guided courses on YouTube, or dozens of classes you can sign up for in your local town, there's no reason why you can't make this a part of your day.

Work yoga in at least 2 times per week, and reap excellent health benefits.

Walking.

Who would have thought that something as simple as walking would be so effective? Yet it is. Just by getting your heart rate up for a few minutes a day is enough to lose some weight.

Set the timer in your house or watch your watch and head outside for a nice walk around the neighborhood. You'll relieve stress and lose weight – it's the best of both worlds.

Jogging.

For those who want to take their weight loss to the next level, try jogging. It's every bit as easy to do as walking, but it boosts your heart rate and gets the blood flowing.

You can do this outside or in the privacy of your own home, just push yourself to go at the safest pace you can, and bring your heartrate up higher than you would with a gentle walk.

Even more stress relieving capabilities here, and you'll look great, too.

Weight lifting.

Weight lifting sounds intimidating, but it doesn't have to be. With just a couple of pounds in each hand as you walk, you maximize your caloric burn while building muscle. Don't get crazy with the weights, get serious about your health.

Chapter 3 – Japanese Diet: Breakfasts

Although not all foods on the Japanese diet are inherently Japanese, the main goal of the diet remains the same. What you are shooting for is a low calorie diet without snacking, and one that also avoids alcohol, sugar, and salt.

Take note that this is added sugar and salt, and those already present in these simple foods is fine. Alcohol is strictly avoided, and bread is only eaten when it is on the menu.

While in many ways dairy is allowed on this kind of diet, you must remember that dairy is also high in fats, and could potentially make it more difficult for you to lose weight. When you are on this simple diet, your goal is to lower your caloric intake as much as possible. This is going to, in turn, maximize your weight loss.

You will find that these recipes call for limited dairy, if any at all. If you so choose to add dairy into your diet during these 2 weeks, keep in mind that you should use smaller portions, and it may interfere with your weight loss goals.

Remember not to snack, but that drinking water between meals is highly important. Drink up to 8 glasses (8 ounces each) of water each day.

Monday – week 1
Simply Buzzed

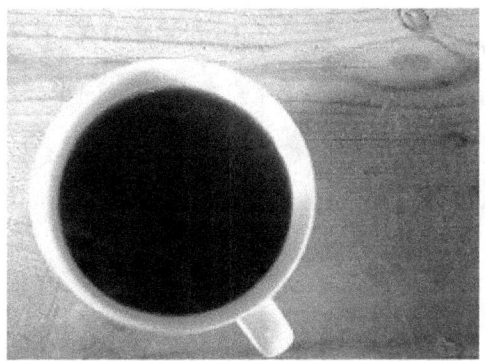

What you will need:

1 eight or ten ounce mug of black coffee

Directions:

Brew the coffee and enjoy black either hot or iced. Drink within 20 minutes.

Tuesday – week 1

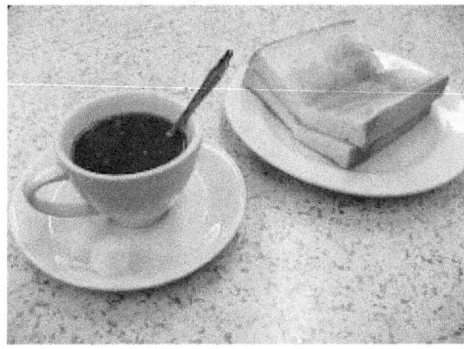

Caffeine and Carbs

What you will need:

1 eight or ten ounce mug of black coffee

1 slice bread, whole grain – no butter

Directions:

Brew the coffee and enjoy black either hot or iced. Drink within 20 minutes.

As the coffee is brewing, toast 1 slice of whole grain bread. Enjoy with your coffee.

Wednesday – week 1

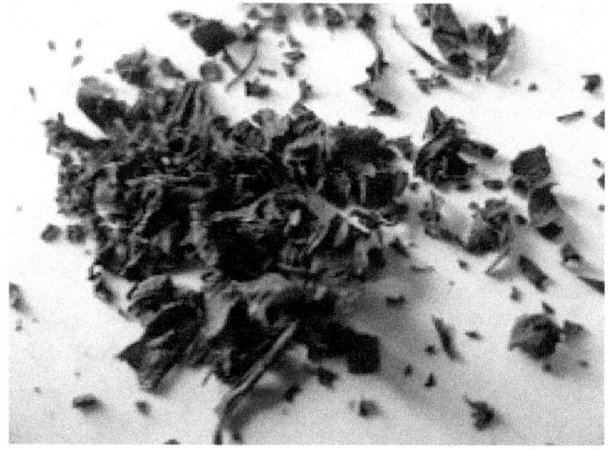

Tiny Power

What you will need:

1 eight or ten ounce mug of black tea

Directions:

Brew the tea and enjoy black either hot or iced. Drink within 20 minutes.

Thursday – week 1
Jack in the Box

What you will need:

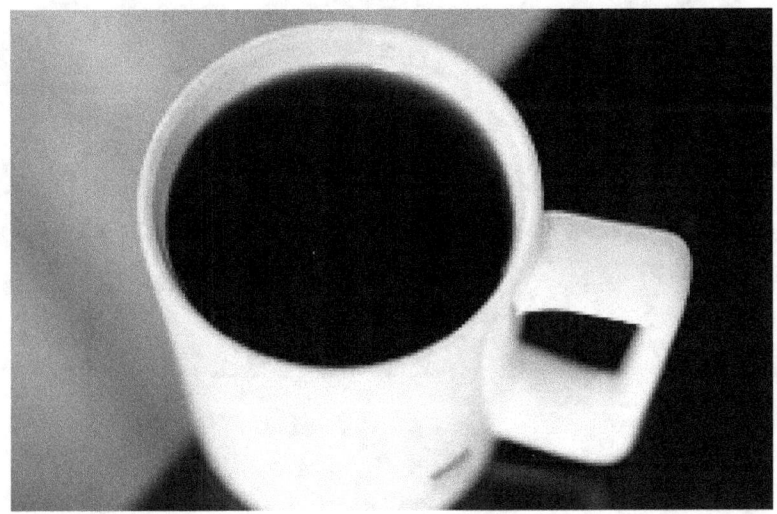

1 eight or ten ounce mug of black coffee

Directions:

Brew the coffee and enjoy black either hot or iced. Drink within 20 minutes.

Friday – week 1
Tea Time

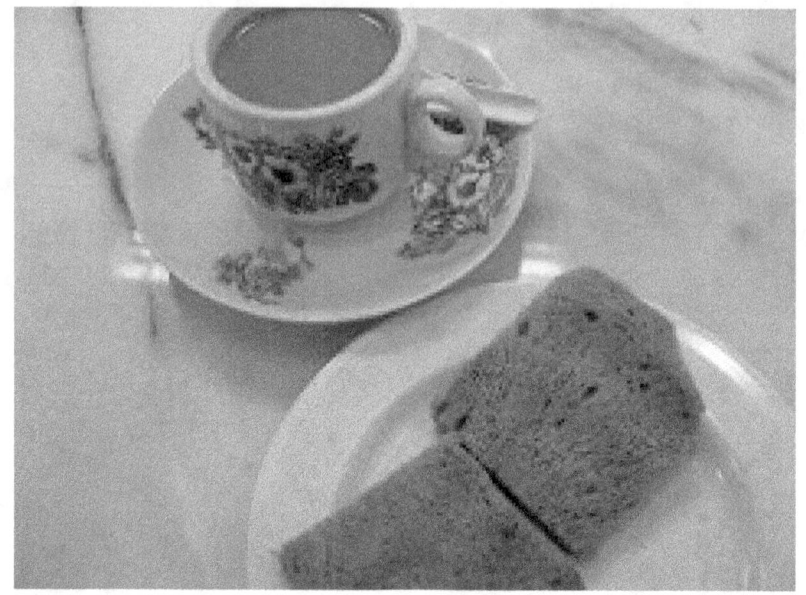

What you will need:

1 eight or ten ounce mug of black tea

1 slice bread, whole grain – no butter

Directions:

Brew the tea and enjoy black either hot or iced. Drink within 20 minutes.

As the tea is brewing, toast 1 slice of whole grain bread. Enjoy with your tea.

Saturday – week 1
The Greener Side

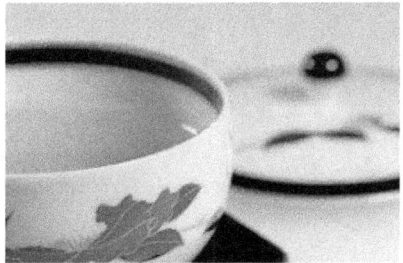

What you will need:

1 eight or ten ounce mug of green tea

Directions:

Brew the tea and enjoy plain either hot or iced. Drink within 20 minutes.

Sunday – week 1
Go Back Black

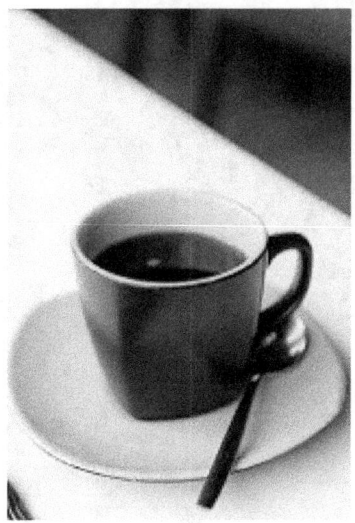

What you will need:

1 eight or ten ounce mug of black coffee

Directions:

Brew the coffee and enjoy black either hot or iced. Drink within 20 minutes.

Monday – week 2
Tea Time Too

What you will need:

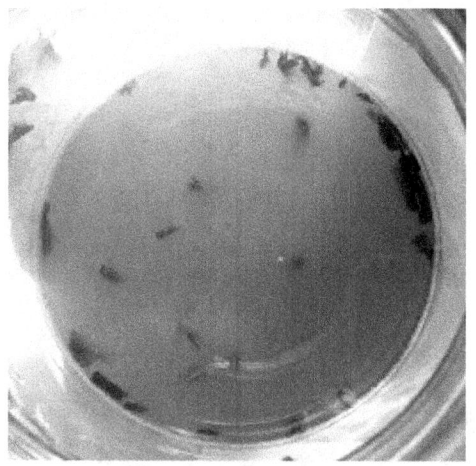

1 eight or ten ounce mug of black tea

Directions:

Brew the tea and enjoy black either hot or iced. Drink within 20 minutes.

Tuesday – week 2

It's a Date

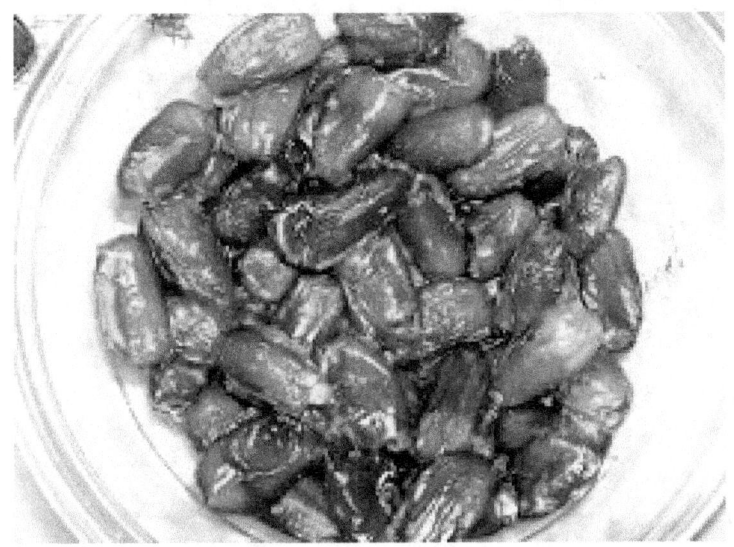

What you will need:

1 eight or ten ounce mug of black coffee

4 dates

Directions:

Brew the coffee and enjoy black either hot or iced. Drink within 20 minutes.

Enjoy the dates with your coffee.

Wednesday – week 2
The Get Up and Go

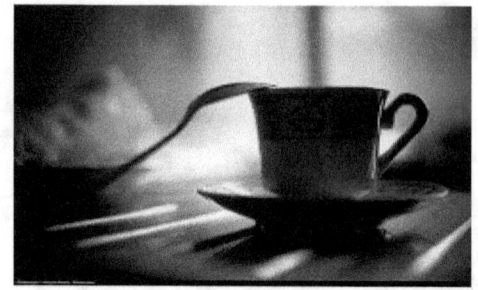

What you will need:

1 eight or ten ounce mug of black coffee

Directions:

Brew the coffee and enjoy black either hot or iced. Drink within 20 minutes.

Thursday – week 2
Goods 'n' Grains

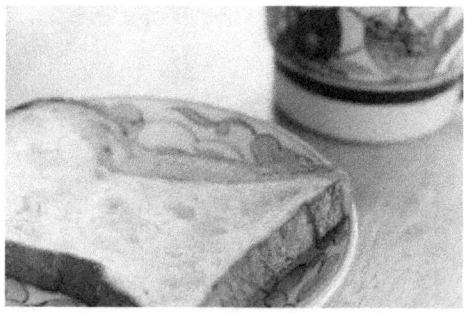

What you will need:

1 eight or ten ounce mug of black coffee

1 slice bread, whole grain – no butter

Directions:

Brew the coffee and enjoy black either hot or iced. Drink within 20 minutes.

As the coffee is brewing, toast 1 slice of whole grain bread. Enjoy with your coffee.

Friday – week 2
The Grass is Greener

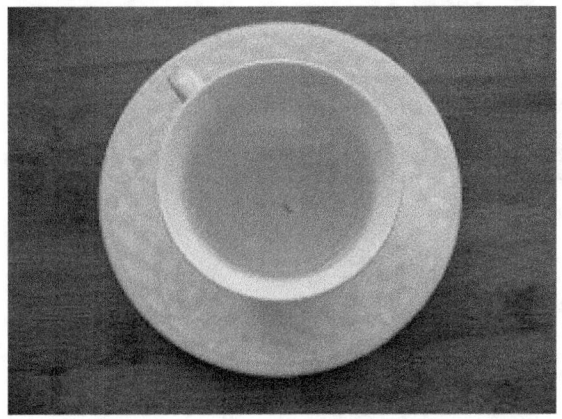

What you will need:

1 eight or ten ounce mug of green tea

Directions:

Brew the tea and enjoy plain either hot or iced. Drink within 20 minutes.

Saturday – week 2
The Fruity Side

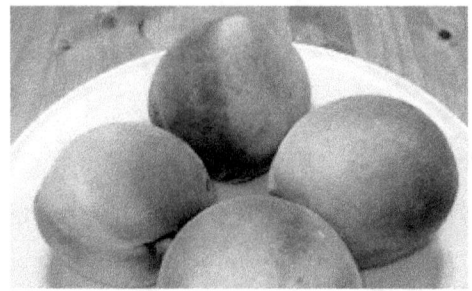

What you will need:

1 eight or ten ounce mug of black coffee

1 peach

Directions:

Brew the coffee and enjoy black either hot or iced. Drink within 20 minutes.

Slice the fruit and enjoy as is with your coffee.

Sunday – week 2
It's All White

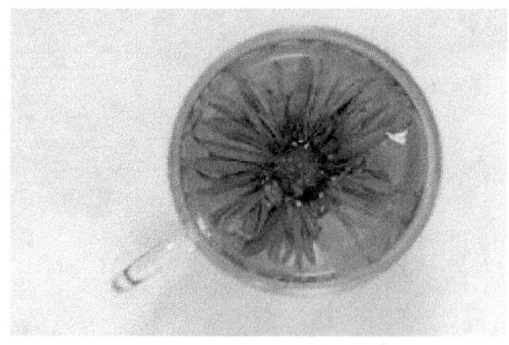

What you will need:

1 eight or ten ounce mug of white tea

Directions:

Brew the tea and enjoy black either hot or iced. Drink within 20 minutes.

Chapter 4 – Japanese Diet: Lunches

Although not all foods on the Japanese diet are inherently Japanese, the main goal of the diet remains the same. What you are shooting for is a low calorie diet without snacking, and one that also avoids alcohol, sugar, and salt.

Take note that this is added sugar and salt, and those already present in these simple foods is fine. Alcohol is strictly avoided, and bread is only eaten when it is on the menu.

While in many ways dairy is allowed on this kind of diet, you must remember that dairy is also high in fats, and could potentially make it more difficult for you to lose weight. When you are on this simple diet, your goal is to lower your caloric intake as much as possible. This is going to, in turn, maximize your weight loss.

You will find that these recipes call for limited dairy, if any at all. If you so choose to add dairy into your diet during these 2 weeks, keep in mind that you should use smaller portions, and it may interfere with your weight loss goals.

Remember not to snack, but that drinking water between meals is highly important. Drink up to 8 glasses (8 ounces each) of water each day.

Monday – week 1
Delicious Egg Salad

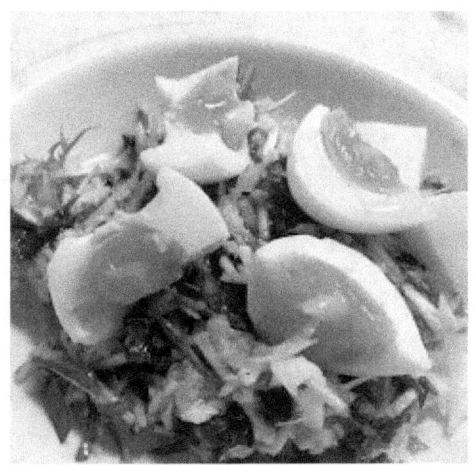

What you will need:

2 hardboiled eggs

1 cup romaine lettuce

1 large tomato

Lemon juice for dressing

Directions:

Start by slicing the eggs into bite sized pieces. Crumble them, if desired.

Wash everything that is going to be a part of the salad and set aside.

Wash the romaine thoroughly, then slice everything to being salad sized. Assemble your salad on a large plate, and spritz with as much lemon juice as you would like.

Add pepper or garlic powder, if desired, but avoid salt as much as possible.

Tuesday – week 1
Mixed Medley

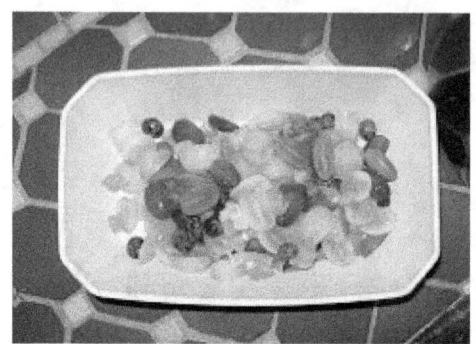

What you will need:

½ cup grapes

1 peach

½ cup strawberries

Directions:

Begin with washing the fruit thoroughly, then slice it into the desired size and shape.

Mix together in a large bowl, and enjoy immediately. Consume within 20 minutes.

Wednesday – week 1
Tuna Tower Power

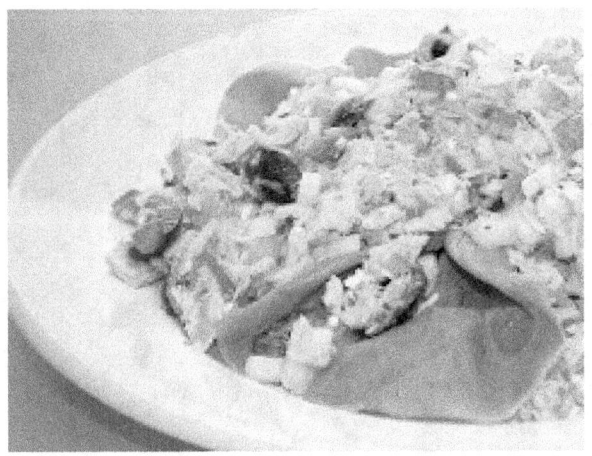

What you will need:

1 can tuna

1 cup romaine lettuce

1 large tomato

Lemon juice for dressing

Directions:

Start by opening and draining the can. You can steam the fish, if desired, or enjoy it as is.

Wash everything that is going to be a part of the salad and set aside.

Wash the romaine thoroughly, then slice everything to being salad sized. Assemble your salad on a large plate, and spritz with as much lemon juice as you would like.

Add pepper or garlic powder, if desired, but avoid salt as much as possible.

Thursday – week 1
It's All in the Rice

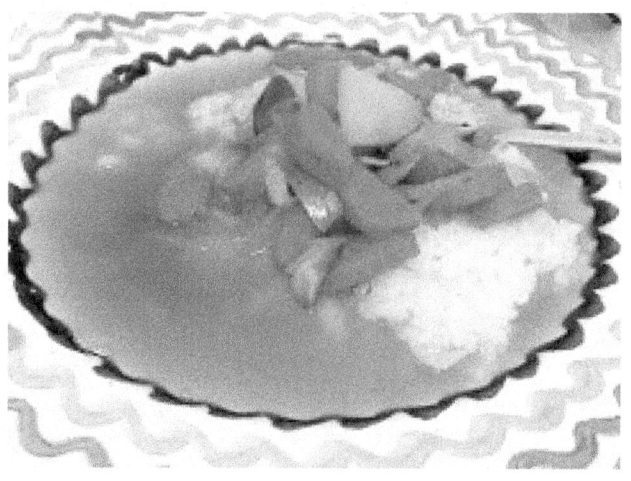

What you will need:

2 carrots

1 teaspoon lemon juice

1 cup cooked rice

Directions:

Coin the carrots and steam them in a vegetable steamer for 10 minutes, until they are soft.

Make sure you are starting with rice that is cooked. If not, bring ¼ cup rice to a boil in ¾ cup water. Cover and allow to simmer for 25 minutes.

Serve with the carrots, garnished with the lemon juice, and pepper, if desired.

Friday – week 1
Best Ever Salmon and Rice

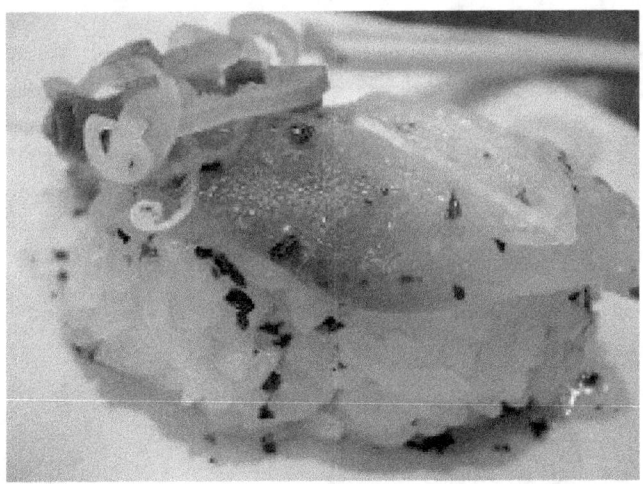

What you will need:

1 small can salmon

1 cup cooked rice

Pepper to taste

Directions:

Start by opening and draining the can. You can steam the fish, if desired, or enjoy it as is.

Make sure you are starting with rice that is cooked. If not, bring ¼ cup rice to a boil in ¾ cup water. Cover and allow to simmer for 25 minutes.

Serve with the salmon, and garnish with pepper, if desired.

Saturday – week 1
Exemplary Avocado Toast

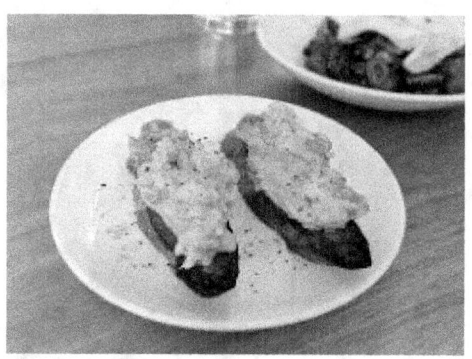

What you will need:

1 avocado

1 slice whole grain bread

Pepper

Garlic

Directions:

Toast the bread on the stove, using a tiny bit of coconut oil. Again, avoid added fats with butter or other dairy. Open and slice the avocado, removing the core.

Spread the avocado onto the bread, seasoning to taste. Avoid salt.

Sunday – week 1
Best Ever Veggie Salad

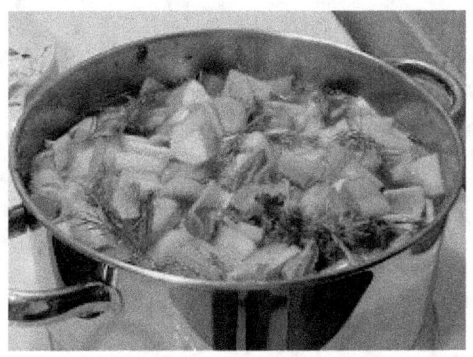

What you will need:

1 cup romaine lettuce

1 carrot

1 large tomato

1 tablespoon lemon juice

Directions:

Wash everything that is going to be a part of the salad and set aside.

Wash the romaine thoroughly, then slice everything to being salad sized. Assemble your salad on a large plate, and spritz with as much lemon juice as you would like.

Add pepper or garlic powder, if desired, but avoid salt as much as possible.

Monday – week 2
Better Than Chicken Salad

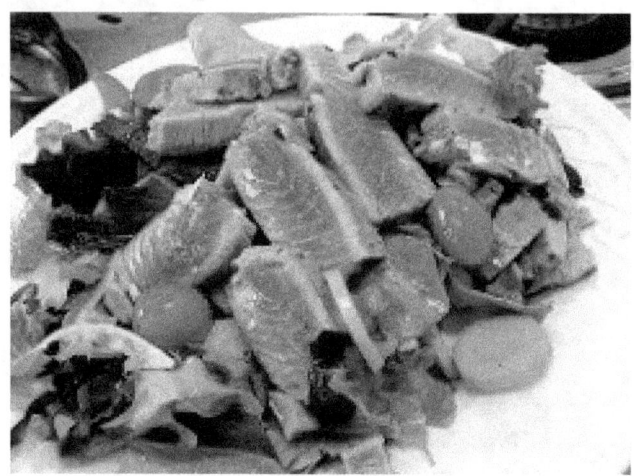

What you will need:

1 can tuna

1 cup romaine lettuce

1 carrot

Lemon juice

Directions:

Start by opening and draining the can. You can steam the fish, if desired, or enjoy it as is.

Wash everything that is going to be a part of the salad and set aside.

Wash the romaine thoroughly, then slice everything to being salad sized. Assemble your salad on a large plate, and spritz with as much lemon juice as you would like.

Add pepper or garlic powder, if desired, but avoid salt as much as possible.

Tuesday – week 2

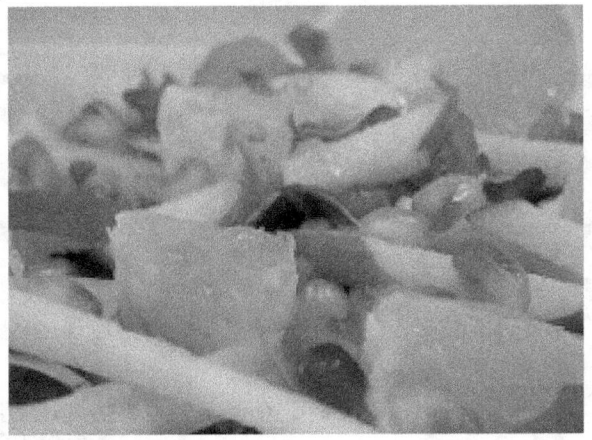

Fruit of the Trees Medley

What you will need:

1 apple

1 peach

1 pear

Directions:

Begin with washing the fruit thoroughly, then slice it into the desired size and shape.

Mix together in a large bowl, and enjoy immediately. Consume within 20 minutes.

Wednesday – week 2
Potato Bake

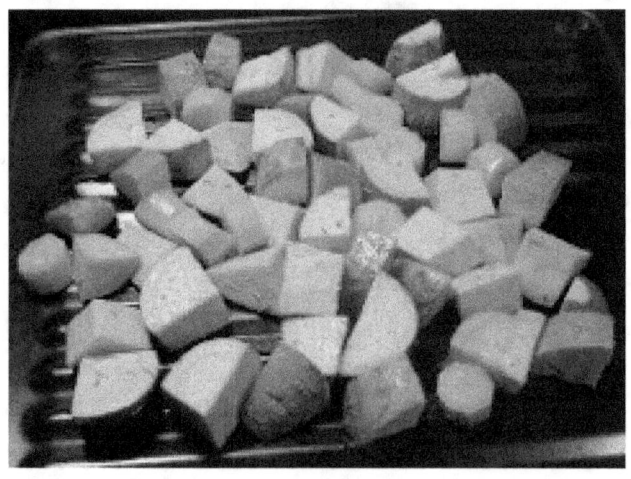

What you will need:

2 large carrots

1 potato

Olive oil

Garlic

Pepper

Directions:

Preheat oven to 350 degrees, and grease a baking sheet with a touch of olive oil. Slice the potato and the carrots, then place them in the oil on this sheet.

Bake for 20 to 30 minutes, stirring halfway through to ensure the potatoes cook thoroughly. Stir and serve immediately.

Thursday – week 2
Not Quite Coleslaw

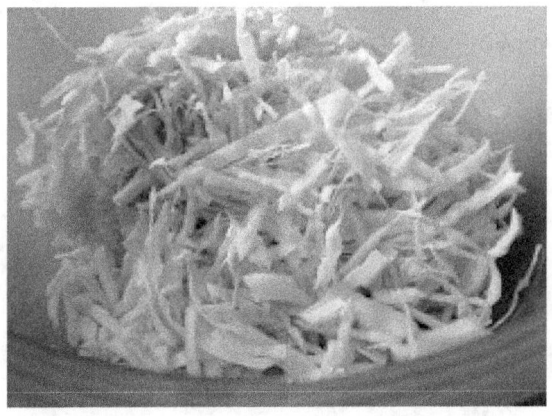

What you will need:

1 cup shredded cabbage

1 shredded carrot

1 stalk celery

Lemon juice

Pepper

Directions:

Wash everything that is going to be a part of the salad and set aside.

Wash the romaine thoroughly, then slice everything to being salad sized. Assemble your salad on a large plate, and spritz with as much lemon juice as you would like.

Add pepper or garlic powder, if desired, but avoid salt as much as possible.

Friday – week 2
Tuna Topped Toast

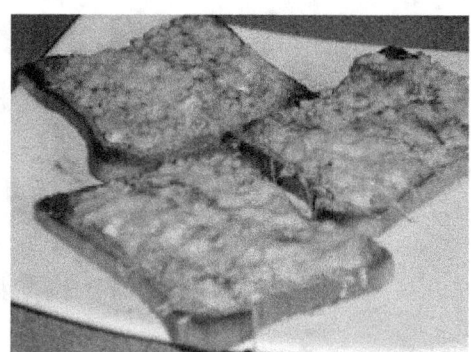

What you will need:

1 can tuna

1 slice bread

1 avocado

Directions:

Start by opening and draining the can. You can steam the fish, if desired, or enjoy it as is.

Toast the bread on the stove, using a tiny bit of coconut oil. Again, avoid added fats with butter or other dairy. Open and slice the avocado, removing the core.

Spread the avocado onto the bread, seasoning to taste. Avoid salt.

Saturday – week 2
The Avocado Rueben

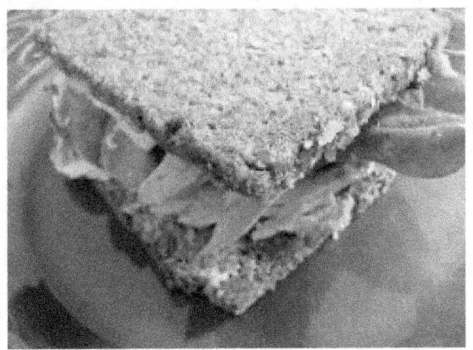

What you will need:

2 slices bread

½ cup sauerkraut

1 avocado

Directions:

Toast the bread on the stove, using a tiny bit of coconut oil. Again, avoid added fats with butter or other dairy. Open and slice the avocado, removing the core.

Add the sauerkraut to the bread on the stove, and continue to cook until it has been heated through.

Spread the avocado onto the bread, that doesn't have the sauerkraut on it, then close as a sandwich, seasoning to taste. Avoid salt.

Sunday – week 2

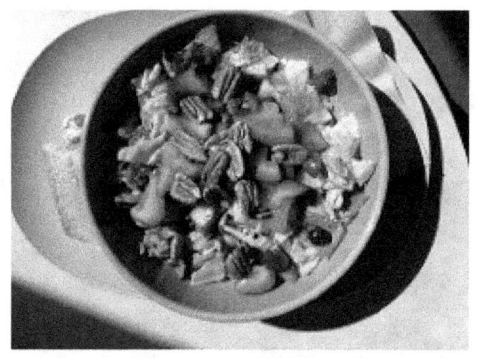

Strawberry Tuna Salad

What you will need:

1 can tuna

½ cup strawberries

1 cup romaine lettuce

Lemon juice

Directions:

Start by opening and draining the can. You can steam the fish, if desired, or enjoy it as is.

Wash everything that is going to be a part of the salad and set aside.

Wash the romaine thoroughly, then slice everything to being salad sized. Assemble your salad on a large plate, and spritz with as much lemon juice as you would like.

Add pepper or garlic powder, if desired, but avoid salt as much as possible.

Enjoy immediately.

Chapter 5 – Japanese Diet: Dinners

Although not all foods on the Japanese diet are inherently Japanese, the main goal of the diet remains the same. What you are shooting for is a low calorie diet without snacking, and one that also avoids alcohol, sugar, and salt.

Take note that this is added sugar and salt, and those already present in these simple foods is fine. Alcohol is strictly avoided, and bread is only eaten when it is on the menu.

While in many ways dairy is allowed on this kind of diet, you must remember that dairy is also high in fats, and could potentially make it more difficult for you to lose weight. When you are on this simple diet, your goal is to lower your caloric intake as much as possible. This is going to, in turn, maximize your weight loss.

You will find that these recipes call for limited dairy, if any at all. If you so choose to add dairy into your diet during these 2 weeks, keep in mind that you should use smaller portions, and it may interfere with your weight loss goals.

Remember not to snack, but that drinking water between meals is highly important. Drink up to 8 glasses (8 ounces each) of water each day.

Monday – week 1
Salmon and Rice Done Right

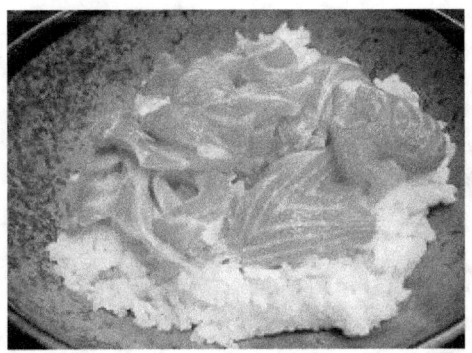

What you will need:

1 cup cooked rice

1 fresh salmon patty

2 carrots

Directions:

Make sure you are starting with cooked rice. You want to have 1 cup cooked rice with your dinner. If your rice isn't cooked, place ¼ - 1/3 cup rice in ¾ to 1 cup water, respectively.

Bring the water to a boil, then simmer on the stove for 25 minutes. You now have 1 cup cooked rice.

Preheat your oven to 350 degrees F, and cook the salmon for 25 minutes, as the rice is cooking if need be.

Coin the carrots, then mix them all together to enjoy.

Tuesday – week 1
Rice Pudding Twist

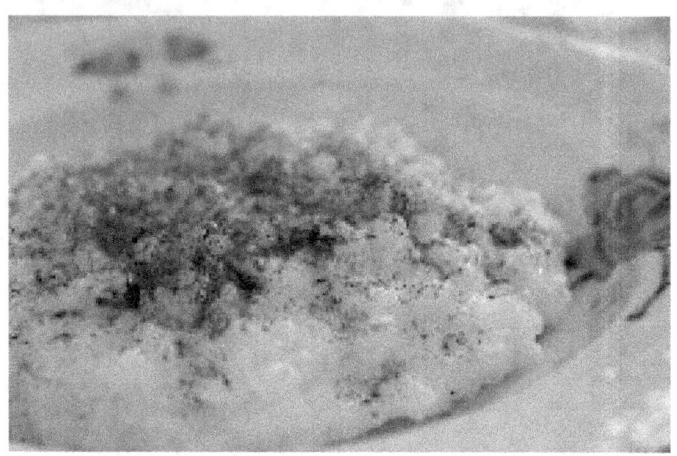

What you will need:

1 cup cooked rice

1 apple

1 teaspoon cinnamon

Directions:

Make sure you are starting with cooked rice. You want to have 1 cup cooked rice with your dinner. If your rice isn't cooked, place ¼ - 1/3 cup rice in ¾ to 1 cup water, respectively.

Bring the water to a boil, then simmer on the stove for 25 minutes. You now have 1 cup cooked rice.

Slice the apple and stir together with the rice and cinnamon. Serve hot or warm.

Wednesday – week 1
Eggs and Rice

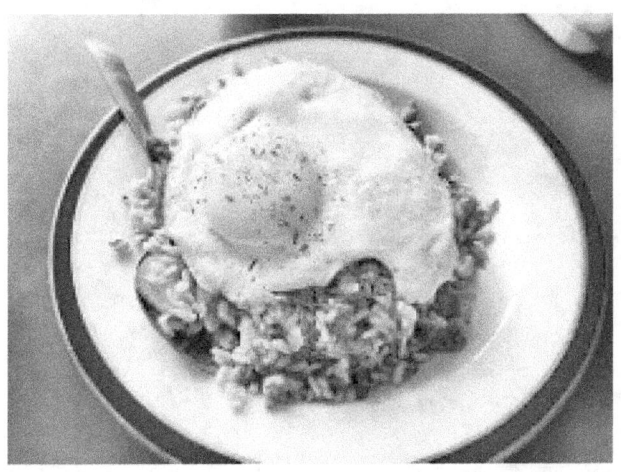

What you will need:

1 cup cooked rice

2 fried eggs

Pepper

Directions:

Make sure you are starting with cooked rice. You want to have 1 cup cooked rice with your dinner. If your rice isn't cooked, place ¼ - 1/3 cup rice in ¾ to 1 cup water, respectively.

Bring the water to a boil, then simmer on the stove for 25 minutes. You now have 1 cup cooked rice.

Fry the eggs in a bit of coconut oil on the stove, then season with pepper and serve with the rice.

Thursday – week 1

Tuna 'n' Rice

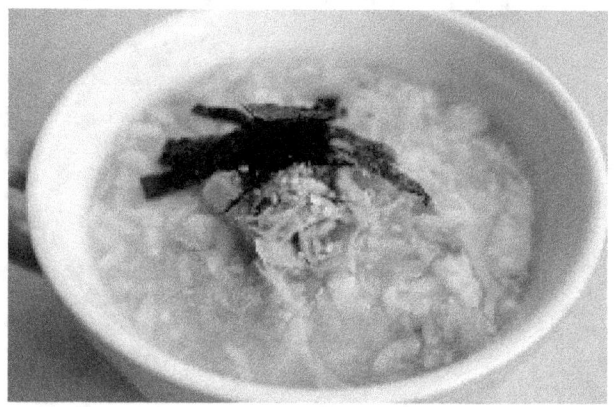

What you will need:

1 cup cooked rice

1 can tuna

1 sliced apple

Directions:

Make sure you are starting with cooked rice. You want to have 1 cup cooked rice with your dinner. If your rice isn't cooked, place ¼ - 1/3 cup rice in ¾ to 1 cup water, respectively.

Bring the water to a boil, then simmer on the stove for 25 minutes. You now have 1 cup cooked rice.

Open and drain the can of tuna, and heat up, if desired. Slice the apple, and combine everything on your plate. Serve warm or hot.

Friday – week 1
Rice Done Right

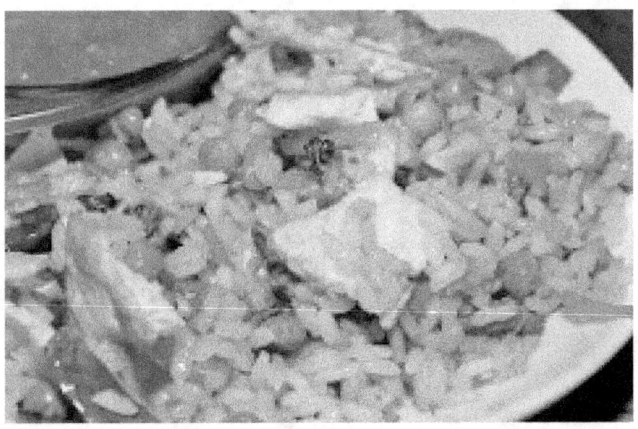

What you will need:

1 cup cooked rice

1 cup peas

1 cup diced carrots

Directions:

Make sure you are starting with cooked rice. You want to have 1 cup cooked rice with your dinner. If your rice isn't cooked, place ¼ - 1/3 cup rice in ¾ to 1 cup water, respectively.

Bring the water to a boil, then simmer on the stove for 25 minutes. You now have 1 cup cooked rice.

Steam the peas with the carrots then mix with the rice. Garnish with pepper or lemon juice, if desired.

Saturday – week 1
The Salmon Rice Twist

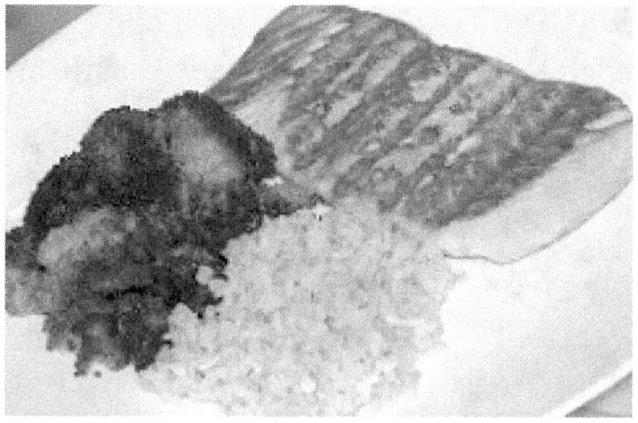

What you will need:

1 cup cooked rice

1 fresh salmon patty

2 stalks celery

Directions:

Make sure you are starting with cooked rice. You want to have 1 cup cooked rice with your dinner. If your rice isn't cooked, place ¼ - 1/3 cup rice in ¾ to 1 cup water, respectively.

Bring the water to a boil, then simmer on the stove for 25 minutes. You now have 1 cup cooked rice.

Preheat your oven to 350 degrees F, and cook the salmon for 25 minutes, as the rice is cooking if need be.

Slice the celery into moons, and mix with the salmon and rice to enjoy.

Sunday – week 1
Now That's Broccoli

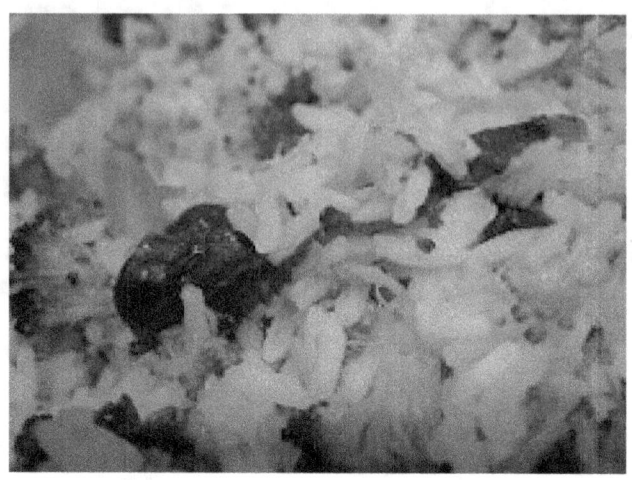

What you will need:

1 cup cooked rice

½ cup broccoli

1 carrot

Directions:

Make sure you are starting with cooked rice. You want to have 1 cup cooked rice with your dinner. If your rice isn't cooked, place ¼ - 1/3 cup rice in ¾ to 1 cup water, respectively.

Bring the water to a boil, then simmer on the stove for 25 minutes. You now have 1 cup cooked rice.

Chop and steam the veggies, then combine with the rice to serve. Garnish with pepper or lemon juice, if desired.

Monday – week 2
Show Me the Steak

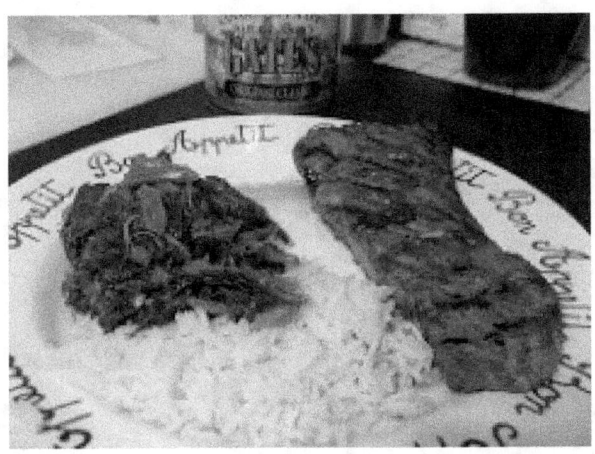

\

What you will need:

1 cup cooked rice

1 small seared steak

Pepper to taste

Directions:

Make sure you are starting with cooked rice. You want to have 1 cup cooked rice with your dinner. If your rice isn't cooked, place ¼ - 1/3 cup rice in ¾ to 1 cup water, respectively.

Bring the water to a boil, then simmer on the stove for 25 minutes. You now have 1 cup cooked rice.

Pan sear the steak so the outside is cooked and the inside is still red. Garnish with the pepper, and serve with rice.

Tuesday – week 2
Doing Things Your Way

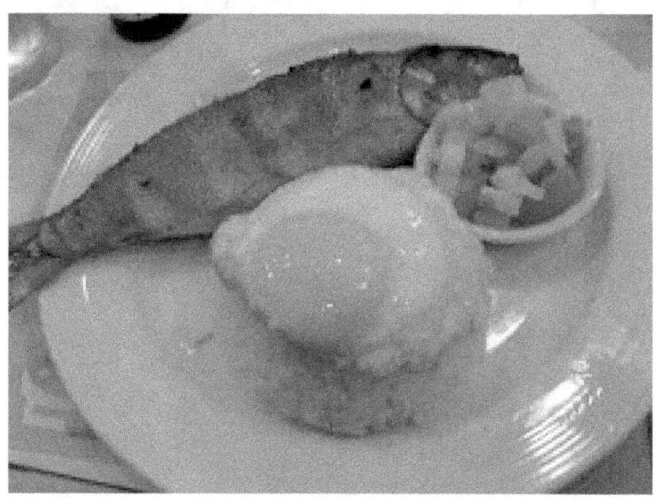

What you will need:

2 eggs, cooked as you like

1 fresh salmon patty

Pepper to taste

Directions:

Make sure you are starting with cooked rice. You want to have 1 cup cooked rice with your dinner. If your rice isn't cooked, place ¼ - 1/3 cup rice in ¾ to 1 cup water, respectively.

Bring the water to a boil, then simmer on the stove for 25 minutes. You now have 1 cup cooked rice.

Preheat your oven to 350 degrees F, and cook the salmon for 25 minutes, as the rice is cooking if need be.

Cook the eggs as you prefer, and serve as a side to the salmon and rice.

Wednesday – week 2
Cauli Fried Rice

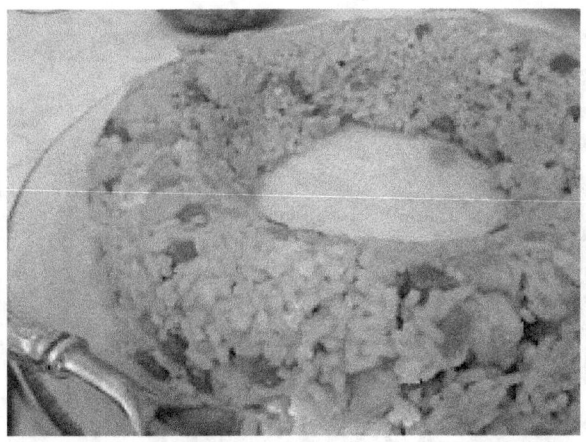

What you will need:

1 cup cooked rice

½ cup minced cauliflower

Pepper to taste

Directions:

Make sure you are starting with cooked rice. You want to have 1 cup cooked rice with your dinner. If your rice isn't cooked, place ¼ - 1/3 cup rice in ¾ to 1 cup water, respectively.

Bring the water to a boil, then simmer on the stove for 25 minutes. You now have 1 cup cooked rice.

Toss everything in a pan on the stove and cook until the cauliflower is cooked through. enjoy immediately.

Thursday – week 2
Chicken of the Sea

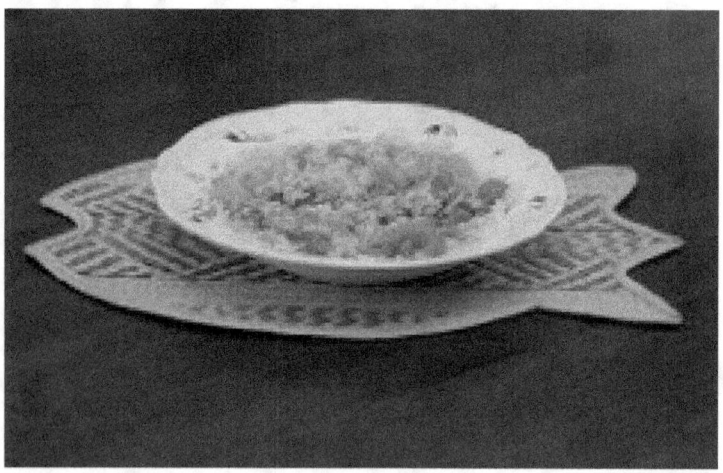

What you will need:

1 cup cooked rice

1 can tuna

Pepper

1 sliced apple

Directions:

Make sure you are starting with cooked rice. You want to have 1 cup cooked rice with your dinner. If your rice isn't cooked, place ¼ - 1/3 cup rice in ¾ to 1 cup water, respectively.

Bring the water to a boil, then simmer on the stove for 25 minutes. You now have 1 cup cooked rice.

Open and drain the can of tuna, steaming it, if desired. Slice the apple, then mix everything together on your plate before serving.

Friday – week 2
Another Way to Veggie

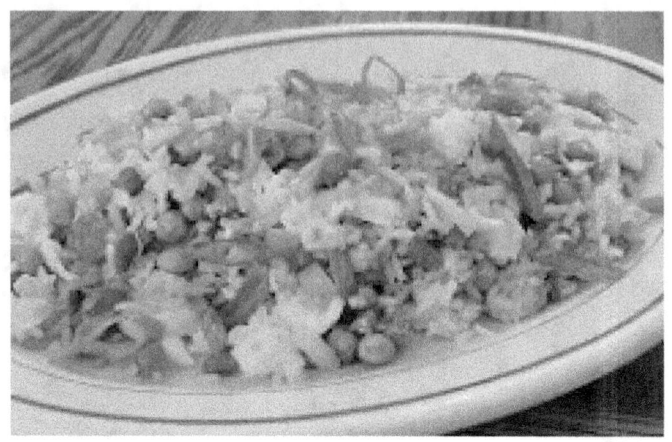

What you will need:

1 cup cooked rice

1 carrot

1 stalk celery

Directions:

Make sure you are starting with cooked rice. You want to have 1 cup cooked rice with your dinner. If your rice isn't cooked, place ¼ - 1/3 cup rice in ¾ to 1 cup water, respectively.

Bring the water to a boil, then simmer on the stove for 25 minutes. You now have 1 cup cooked rice.

Slice the steam the veggies, then stir them together with your rice and enjoy. Garnish with lemon juice or pepper, if desired.

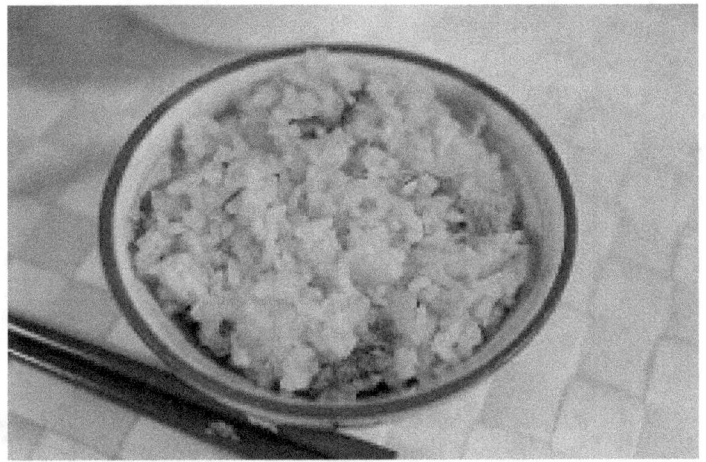

Salmon Meets Peas

What you will need:

1 cup cooked rice

1 can salmon

1 cup peas

Directions:

Make sure you are starting with cooked rice. You want to have 1 cup cooked rice with your dinner. If your rice isn't cooked, place ¼ - 1/3 cup rice in ¾ to 1 cup water, respectively.

Bring the water to a boil, then simmer on the stove for 25 minutes. You now have 1 cup cooked rice.

Open and drain the can of salmon, heating if desired. Stir all ingredients together, and enjoy hot or warm.

Sunday – week 2
Crunch Time

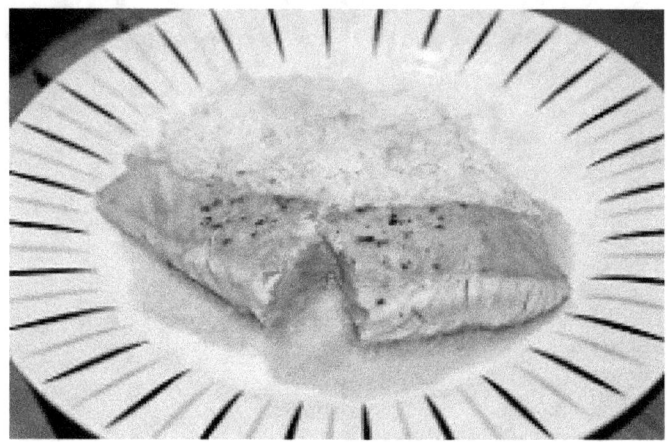

What you will need:

1 cup cooked rice

1 fresh salmon patty

2 celery stalks

Directions:

Make sure you are starting with cooked rice. You want to have 1 cup cooked rice with your dinner. If your rice isn't cooked, place ¼ - 1/3 cup rice in ¾ to 1 cup water, respectively.

Bring the water to a boil, then simmer on the stove for 25 minutes. You now have 1 cup cooked rice.

Preheat your oven to 350 degrees F, and cook the salmon for 25 minutes, as the rice is cooking if need be.

Layer with the celery, but leave the celery raw. Enjoy immediately.

Conclusion

There you have it, everything you need to get started on the Japanese diet, and to lose 15 pounds in as little as two weeks. I hope this book was able to give you the inspiration you need to get started on a weight loss journey, and to lose weight.

You're going to find with this diet that it is easier than ever to lose the weight you want to lose, and get healthy. Remember to follow both the rules of the diet, and to listen to your own body. With any fast diets, there are some risks to be aware of, but if you listen to what your body is telling you, you aren't going to have any problems.

Now get out there and lose the weight you want to lose. Summer is just around the corner, and you need to be ready for it.

Good luck.

FREE Bonus Reminder

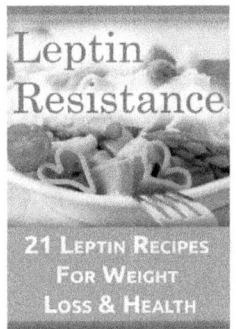

If you have not grabbed it yet, please go ahead and download your special bonus report *"Leptin Resistance. 21 Leptin Recipes For Weight Loss & Healthy Living"*.

Simply Click the Button Below

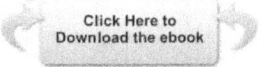

OR **Go to This Page**

http://easyweightlossway.com/free/

BONUS #2: More Free Books

Do you want to receive more Free Books?

We have a mailing list where we send out our new Books when they go free on Kindle. Click on the link below to sign up for Free Book Promotions. => Sign Up for Free Book Promotions <=

OR Go to this URL http://bit.ly/1V4Xan7